MW00441460

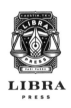

LIBRA

PRESS

THE TRIP JOURNAL

ISBN 978-1-955858-08-3

DESIGN BY FLORENCIA BALDINI AND ERIN TYLER. COVER AND
ILLUSTRATIONS BY ERIN TYLER. PRINTED IN THE USA.

TRIPJOURNAL.CO

The Trip Journal

CREATED BY

Ronan Levy and Kori Harrison

IF FOUND, PLEASE CONTACT

_____

_____

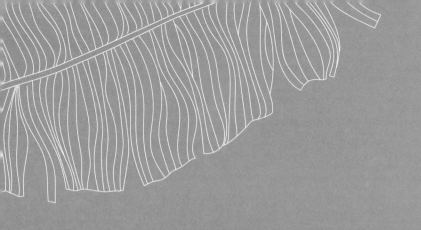

Your vision will become clear only
when you can look into your own
heart. Who looks outside, dreams;
who looks inside, awakes.

–CARL JUNG

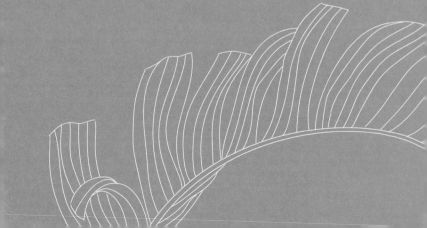

DEDICATION

To those with the courage to look inward with
open humility. That is true strength. A simple act
makes the world a better place.

Contents

· ·

Foreword

BY ANDREW WEIL, MD

Psychedelic journeying can be immensely rewarding, a great assist to personal growth and development. But just taking psilocybin, LSD, or MDMA does not guarantee a positive experience. Early in my research on these and other psychoactive substances, including cannabis, I learned that their effects were products not just of pharmacology but of interactions with other factors. What people commonly call "drug effects" are, in fact, the combined effects of drug, set, and setting.

"Drug" means the pharmacological nature of the substance, the dose, and the route of administration. "Set" denotes the expectations, both conscious and unconscious, of the person taking it. "Setting" is the environment, both physical and cultural, in which it is taken. The combined influence of set and setting can greatly modify, even reverse, pharmacological action.

Under certain conditions of set and setting, a person taking a stimulant might fall asleep; one taking a sedative might become agitated.

The experiences of psychedelic journeyers are especially shaped by set and setting. When I was an undergraduate at Harvard in 1960, I knew several students who were dosed with LSD at a party without their knowledge. Like most people at that time, they had never heard of LSD. When they felt its pharmacological effects, they interpreted them as food poisoning. They had no expectations of a psychedelic journey and no support from the party setting to go on one.

Compare that with the many reports of people having full-blown psychedelic experiences after taking placebos. A 2020 study reported that more than 60 percent of subjects given an inactive product but told they were given psilocybin felt they were tripping.

In the 1960s, LSD was used experimentally and successfully in terminal cancer patients to help them with the dying process. The researchers had personal experience with LSD. They prepared each patient with several sessions of psychotherapy before their trip and helped them integrate the journey in follow-up sessions.

Afterward, most patients reported decreased fear of death and reduced pain. They required less pain medication and were able to be more present with family and friends—all good outcomes.

Early enthusiasm for the therapeutic potential of LSD waned, however, when other investigators who had no personal experience with the drug and poor understanding of the importance of set and setting tried to reproduce these experiments without success.

The main takeaway is that you must pay careful

attention to all the factors that shape a psychedelic journey. If you take too high a dose of psilocybin or LSD on a day when you feel anxious or depressed, in the company of others who are anxious or depressed, in a non-supportive setting, you are likely to have a bad trip.

For a positive experience, use the right amount of the appropriate substance after you have made proper preparations, including setting an intention for the trip. Make sure you are comfortable with the setting. Especially if it's your first time, I strongly recommend relying on an experienced guide to help navigate the novel terrain that will open to you.

Among Native American peoples who use psychedelic plants, shamans are the guides. They know the terrain thoroughly and are fully competent to help the less experienced through rough patches and get the most out of journeys. Our society does not have shamans, but I am pleased that Field Trip and other organizations are now training health professionals to be psychedelic guides and therapists.

This journal will help you get the most out of all consciousness-expanding activities, not only psychedelic trips but also breathwork, meditation, and more. Writing about these experiences is a sure way to capture their value, integrate them into your life, and draw on them to improve physical, mental, and spiritual well-being.

May you have wonderful journeys!

—*Andrew Weil, MD*

Who this is for

This journal was written for those who are currently working with, or would like to begin working with, consciousness-expanding practices.

These practices can include psychedelic journeying, breathwork, plant medicine, meditation, intensive yoga, cryotherapy, craniosacral therapy, or many other modalities that deepen your self-awareness and empower personal growth.

This book provides you with a carefully constructed process to capture and record your experiences, in order to best learn and grow from them.

Our hope is that it will become an essential companion for all of your trips, providing you with a friend and touchstone along your journeys in expanding your mind and opening your heart.

Disclaimer

Nothing in this book should be viewed as encouraging or inducing you to seek, attain, or procure anything that is illegal in the jurisdictions in which you reside.

Psychedelic experiences can be achieved through a number of legal techniques, such as meditation, breathwork, and use of medically prescribed drugs, such as ketamine, in controlled circumstances with appropriate supervision. There are some herbs and natural products that are known to induce psychedelic-like experiences, and some commonly known psychedelics, like psilocybin mushrooms, are legal in certain jurisdictions.

Please know the laws where you live and follow them appropriately. Also, of course, make sure you understand the risks of anything you do and any substance you take into your body.

All information is provided for informational and educational purposes only and is not intended to be a substitute for medical, mental health, or legal advice under any circumstance. Always consult your primary care physician, other qualified healthcare provider(s), or legal counsel, as appropriate, prior to seeking to participate in any consciousness-expanding practice including but not limited to manufacture, cultivation, or procurement, and prior to using any psychedelic or psychoactive substance, including for treatment of a medical condition. Never disregard professional advice or fail to seek it.

Who we are

RONAN LEVY

Ronan is a lawyer-turned-entrepreneur and visionary with a penchant for questioning paradigms and convention, and in their place seeking truth and impact. A husband, father of two boys, and repeated executive and founder of leading companies in the cannabis and psychedelic industries—including Field Trip Health Ltd.—Ronan's ten-plus-year internal growth journey has been paramount in staying centered and balanced while executing on a groundbreaking vision to change the landscape of mental health. From this journey, one lesson he's internalized is the beauty in seeing life through fresh eyes, like that of a curious child, and he hopes to extend that lens to all and bring the world to life through Field Trip psychedelic therapies and technology.

KORI HARRISON

Kori is a lifelong learner, technologist, investor, and writer. From corporate consulting in DC to building technology startups in Silicon Valley, her mental health and journeys inward weren't a priority for many years. A disciplined soul with an incessant craving for progress, she found consciousness-expanding practices at a time when softening and reframing narratives were especially needed. The improved well-being and self-discoveries she experienced with this work inspired a mission to help others find the same. This brought her to Field Trip, where Kori served as Head of Product leading Field Trip's digital strategy to scaling psychedelic therapies globally. To learn more about her personal journey, visit www.koriharrison.com.

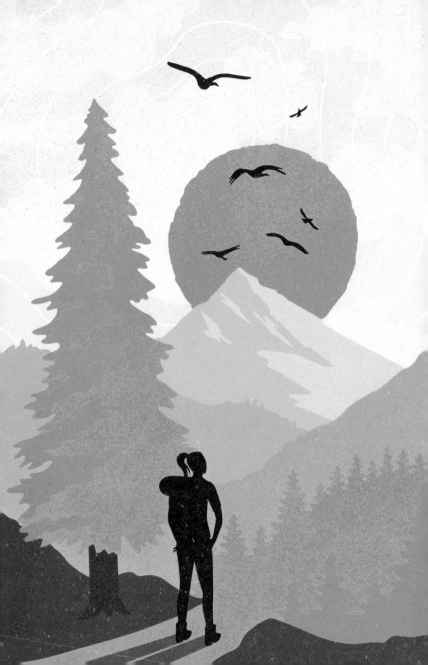

All that you seek is inside you.
It is the process of discovering
that, then letting it be seen,
that liberates.

-UNKNOWN

What is a psychedelic experience?

Commonly referred to as a "trip"

For thousands of years, cultures have used psychedelics as sacramental tools for religious rituals and to connect with a sense of spirituality.

In fact, the word *psychedelic* is the union of "psyche," which means breath, life, soul, or spirit, and "delic," which is derived from delos, meaning "clear, manifest." A psychedelic experience occurs when there is a clearing or manifestation of the mind or spirit.

We define "trip" as any experience that can help you expand your mind from its everyday way of thinking and get an honest look at the way in which you see and make sense of the world, allowing you to uncover aspects of your life or ways of thinking that don't serve you and invite new ways to connect more deeply to yourself, others, and your environment.

What happens when we trip?

The neuroscience and psychology behind psychedelic experiences

W hile there are many studies on this topic currently underway and more to come, research has thus far revealed that the power of psychedelic experiences to promote mental wellness and healing are the result of their ability to temporarily suspend the Default Mode Network (DMN) of the brain (Palhano-Fontes et al. 2015).[1]

The DMN is a section of correlated parts of the brain, consisting primarily of the prefrontal cortex (PFC), posterior cingulate cortex (PCC), and the inferior parietal lobe (IPL).

As the brain matures, the DMN starts to rely more consistently on certain pathways and

1. Palhano-Fontes, Fernanda et. al. 2015. "The Psychedelic State Induced by Ayahuasca Modulates the Activity and Connectivity of the Default Mode Network." Edited by Dewen Hu. PLOS ONE 10, no. 2 (February). https://doi.org/10.1371/journal.pone.0118143.

algorithms that become habitual. This is our brain's way of optimizing energy consumption, by helping us to think more efficiently. This certainly has its benefits, but it also makes learning new behaviors or changing habits more challenging.

The DMN is also thought to be responsible for our ego (Carhart-Harris et al, 2014).[2] According to Sigmund Freud's Personality Theory (Freud 1923),[3] the personality is composed of three elements: the id, the ego, and the superego. The id consists of our primal desires and urges, while the superego is the moral compass that operates from internalized rules we acquire from our caregivers and society. The ego is the mediator between the urges of the id, the idealistic standards of the superego, and the demands of reality. The ego, then, forms the identity that helps us best fit in the world—it defines who

2. Carhart-Harris, Robin L et al. 2014. "The entropic brain: a theory of conscious states informed by neuroimaging research with psychedelic drugs." *Frontiers in Human Neuroscience*, 8, no. 20 (February). doi.org/10.3389/fnhum.2014.00020

3. Freud, Sigmund, et. al. 1961. *The Ego and the Id and Other Works (The Standard Edition of the Completed Psychological Works of Sigmund Freud, Volume XIX [1923 - 1925])*. London: Hogarth Press.

we are to ourselves and how we project ourselves to others. We need an ego to function productively and collaboratively, but when we begin to internalize it, when our ego becomes one and the same with "I," our emotions get wrapped up in maintaining it. This leads to pain, fear, or shame when the ego is bruised, and we form protective, often limiting, walls to avoid that sort of pain in the future. Experiments using functional magnetic resonance imaging (fMRI) and magnetoencephelography (MAG) have shown that during a psychedelic experience—where it is believed "ego dissolution" occurs—the DMN also shuts down temporarily (Millière et al. 2018).[4] This suspension of the DMN allows access to parts of the brain and functions that are not typically used and, as a result, helps our consciousness access new perspectives.

Through the lens of psychology, psychedelic experiences suspend the ego's grip, enabling you to get an objective

4. Millière, Raphaël et. al. 2018. "Psychedelics, Meditation, and Self-Consciousness." *Frontiers in Psychology*, 9. doi.org/10.3389/fpsyg.2018.01475

view on your current definition of self, thus creating an opportunity for change (Nichols 2016).[5] In other words, it helps you get out of your own way.

It is within your power to rewire your brain—to reframe old patterns, or even identities, that don't serve you and build new ones that do. Psychedelic experiences are one path, perhaps a shorter one than conventional methods, to help you do so, and there is a growing body of research that provides insight into how and why.

5. Nichols, David E. 2016. "Psychedelics." *Pharmacological Reviews* 68 (2): 264-355. doi.org/10.1124/pr.115.011478

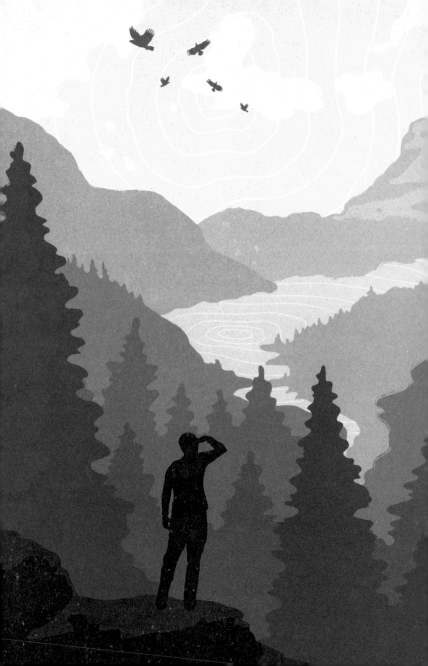

Knowing others is intelligence;
knowing yourself is true wisdom.
Mastering others is strength;
mastering yourself is true power.

-TAO TE CHING

The research on psychedelic experiences

Whatever the route to having a psychedelic experience, there is a compelling amount of evidence that their therapeutic potential far exceeds what has been achievable through conventional psychiatric medications and therapies alone. In the following pages, we'll share a few examples of methods known to induce consciousness expansion and the research on the potential benefits.

Classic psychedelics

As many classic psychedelics, such as LSD, psilocybin, DMT, and mescaline, are controlled substances, we cannot and do not advocate that you use these for your psychedelic experiences.

Some clinical trials have been granted approval to assess the efficacy of a synthetic form of psilocybin, and the results of these studies demonstrate that it holds great promise in treating mental health conditions such as depression and anxiety.

Professor David Nutt regarded the results of the psilocybin depression studies as "remarkable," noting that "two experiences with psilocybin improved depression scores for weeks, and in some people, years positioning it as one of the most powerful therapies for treatment-resistant depression" (Carhart-Harris et al. 2018).[6]

It is believed that the reason for the lasting effects of psychedelics is a therapeutic window following the experience where there is a certain increased malleability in the brain that enables new insights and emotional release that, with psychotherapeutic support, can result in a subsequent healthy revision of one's outlook and lifestyle (Carhart-Harris et al. 2017).[7]

6. Carhart-Harris, Robin L, et al. 2018. "Psilocybin with psychological support for treatment-resistant depression: six-month follow-up." *Psychopharmacology*, 235 (February): 399–408. https://doi.org/10.1007/s00213-017-4771-x

7. Carhart-Harris, RL, et al. 2017. "Psilocybin for treatment-resistant depression: FMRI-measured brain mechanisms." *Scientific Reports* 7 (October). doi.org/10.1038/s41598-017-13282-7

More studies are coming, some now underway, that investigate the use of the classic psychedelic molecules for many mental health issues, including but not limited to PTSD, major depression disorder, treatment-resistant depression, Alzheimer's, attention deficit disorder, anorexia, obsessive compulsive disorder, addiction, and cluster headaches.

Breathwork

There have been a number of studies that have assessed the biological effect and associated therapeutic benefits of different breathing techniques.

Our vagus nerve (Gerritsen et al. 2018)[8] is responsible for the function of our lungs, heart, and diaphragm and controls our states of fight-or-flight versus rest-and-digest. Simply extending exhales to be longer than inhales can help

8 Gerritsen, Roderik JS and Guido PH Band. 2018. "Breath of Life: The Respiratory Vagal Stimulation Model of Contemplative Activity." *Frontiers in Human Neuroscience*, 12: 397. doi.org/10.3389/fnhum.2018.00397

redirect it from a state of hyperarousal back to stable, routine functioning.

One study looking at yoga breathing techniques found a significant reduction in PTSD symptoms (Kim et al. 2013),[9] and the work of the leading expert in PTSD, Dr. Bessel van der Kolk, details the positive effects of yoga (van der Kolk 2014) and pranayama (breathwork) on PTSD and trauma.[10]

Another expert examined a breathing-based meditative technique called Sudarshan Kriya (Sharma et al., 2017) yoga, which resulted in a decrease in depression and anxiety scores.[11]

Holotropic Breathwork

9. Kim, Sang Hwan et. al. 2013. "PTSD symptom reduction with mindfulness-based stretching and deep breathing exercise: randomized controlled clinical trial of efficacy." *Journal of Clinical Endocrinology & Metabolism*, 98 (7): 2984-92. doi.org/10.1210/jc.2012-3742

10. Van der Kolk, Bessel. 2014. "Learning to Inhabit Your Body: Yoga." In *The Body Keeps the Score: Brain, Mind, and Body in the Healing of Trauma*, 263-76. London: Penguin Random House UK.

11. Sharma, Anup et. al. 2017. "A Breathing-Based Meditation Intervention for Patients With Major Depressive Disorder Following Inadequate Response to Antidepressants: A Randomized Pilot Study." *Journal of Clinical Psychiatry*, 78 (1): e59-e63. doi.org/10.4088/JCP.16m10819

(Holmes et al. 1996)[12] is a technique developed by Dr. Stanislov Grof that has been shown to induce a psychedelic-like experience. It's been demonstrated that in combination with experientially oriented verbal psychotherapy, Dr. Grof's methods may facilitate reductions in death anxiety and increases in self-esteem, both of which transpersonal theory posits as the root of seemingly intractable psychological problems.

Meditation

Meditation refers to a set of cognitive techniques and practices that aim to monitor and regulate attention, perception, and emotions.

A breadth of meditation techniques have been developed in many different cultures and spiritual traditions,

12. Holmes, Sara W et. al. 1996. "Holotropic Breathwork: An Experiential Approach to Psychotherapy." *Psychotherapy: Theory, Research, Practice, Training*, 33(1): 114–120. doi.org/10.1037/0033-3204.33.1.114

yielding more than 100 different varieties of meditation. It can be a powerful practice in preparing for, integrating, or even inducing a psychedelic experience.

Research seeking to correlate the neural effects from the varieties of meditation practices known today has come to be known as contemplative neuroscience. The data from these studies has shown that meditation can modulate brain activity in different ways, so we recommend experimenting with at least a few different practices to discover what most resonates with you.

The observed therapeutic benefits of meditation are extensive and last beyond the time in meditation, spanning from objectively improving physical biomarkers related to stress (such as inflammation) to subjectively enhancing mental health and well-being and guiding us back from the mind wandering (Brewer et al. 2011) that our brain naturally does when not focused on a task.[13]

13. Brewer, Judson A et. al. 2011. "Meditation experience is associated with differences in default mode network activity and connectivity." *Proceedings of the National Academy of Sciences of the United States of America*, 108(50): 20254-20259. doi.org/10.1073/pnas.1112029108

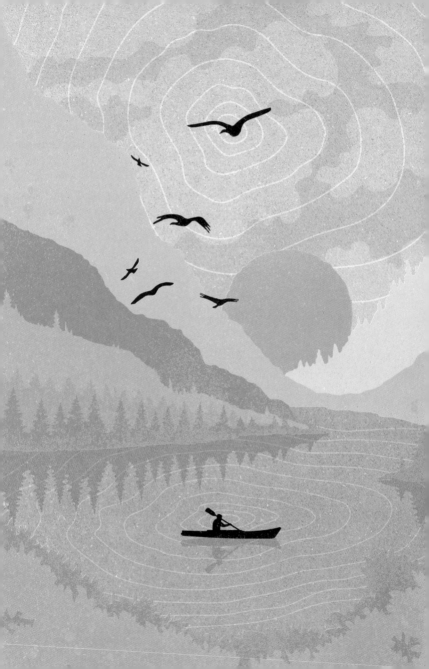

Why write about your experiences?

Y ou've probably heard the cliché that the pen is mightier than the sword, but when it comes to many aspects of our mental and neurological health, the pen is also far mightier than the device.

Writing down the experience of traumatic events has been shown to help speed the emotional and even physical processing that result from those events. This is relevant to this guide because following psychedelic experiences, many people report a changed or better understanding of traumatic events. This new lens with which the traumatic episode is viewed, when paired with the act of writing it down, helps you process the impact of a trauma upon your life and change your outlook for the future.

And there is ample science to confirm this. James Pennebaker, the famed researcher and psychologist at the University of Texas at Austin, has led hundreds of studies over thirty years that have found that the act of writing about your feelings, emotions, and thoughts on paper can:

- Trigger neural activity in the brain, similar to meditation.
- Reduce stress.
- Improve mood, over both the short term and long term.
- Improve performance at school and work.
- Improve almost all measurable markers of social life and happiness.
- Improve immune system function.
- Lower blood pressure.
- Improve sleep.
- Improve markers of chronic illness.
- Increase white blood cell counts in AIDS patients.

- Improve markers of health in cancer patients.

- And dozens more similar results.

This is research only on writing and journaling about thoughts and feelings. For purposes of this guide, the act of writing something down, particularly a psychedelic experience, has two additional key benefits:

First, it helps encode an idea or thought into your brain. Encoding is the process by which the things we perceive travel to our brain's hippocampus, where they are analyzed and ultimately stored in long-term memory. It invites the possibility for changing habitual thinking patterns of the default mode network (DMN). By writing down the details of your psychedelic experience and the insights that you want to take into your future, you greatly improve the potential for those changes to be sustained and integrate into your life.

Second, and perhaps most importantly, keeping a record of trip details such as location, time, and amount helps you calibrate for future journeys.

Psychedelic experiences are generally safe and positive, but challenging feelings and emotions may arise, so it is recommended to keep a clear record of what you are experiencing, when, and what factors surround it so you can best calibrate future sessions.

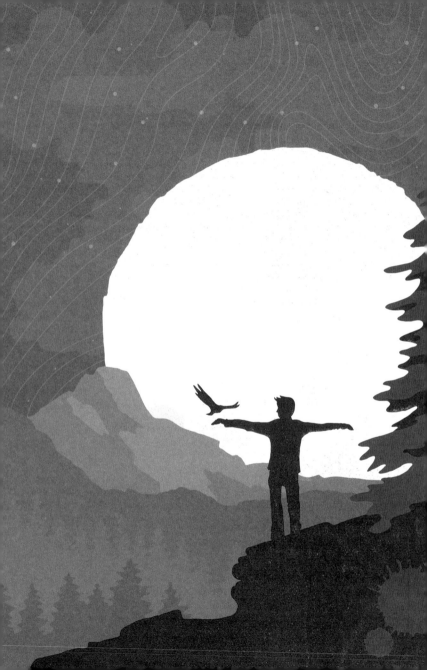

How to use *The Trip Journal*

Each Trip Journal covers ten trips. Each trip has Before, During, and After sections.

The Before Trip section guides you in recording key aspects of your trip for your reference to use as a baseline as you calibrate the approach and setting that works best for you.

The During Trip section is purely optional. Some people like to doodle or take notes during their trip, and this section has no lines for that purpose—to make free flow and association easier.

The After Trip sections are broken down into Days 1 through 5, Day 7, and Day 14.

The format has been carefully crafted and the design thoughtfully laid out to maximize its impact, so it is best to try to follow the processes described as closely as possible. The only deviation would come if you have more to write than the pages can contain.

Preparation:
What to do before your trip

SELECT YOUR SETTING

Select the location where you'll have your psychedelic experience thoughtfully. There is substantial evidence that the setting of an experience can have a material impact on its quality and therapeutic potential. We recommend seeking an environment in which you feel safe, calm, and comfortable throughout the entirety of your planned trip.

RECORD KEEPING

Record the details of your psychedelic experience, such as the location, date, and time, for future reference and tracking. If you are using a prescribed medicine, such as ketamine or another legal herb or product, record the details of the compound and the amounts.

Recording this information will help you calibrate and better prepare for future experiences.

An intention is a purpose or goal around which you want to center your experience. Beyond the physical setting of your planned psychedelic experience, the intention you bring into the experience can impact the quality of your result.

The most therapeutic trips tend to result from beginning with a specific, clear intention that is unique to you.

Examples of intentions could be:

- Processing a past experience, whether positive or negative, traumatic, or empowering, to better understand its purpose in your life and what to learn from it.

- Unveiling and healing pain you may be holding and expressing in unconscious ways.

- Reframing your self-perceptions and narrative identity.

- Letting down walls that hold you back from connecting deeply with yourself and others.

- Understanding the roots under a certain pattern of behavior.

- Overcoming a negative habit or addiction.

- Wanting to feel certain emotions more deeply.

- Releasing feelings that you've held onto, such as hurt, anger, loss, or unrequited love.

For the reasons we already discussed with regard to the power of journaling, it is important to write down your intention(s). In the Trip Journal, we include space to provide context about your intention and your associated feelings, emotions, and memories.

SELECT YOUR MUSIC

Music can have a significant effect on your psychedelic experience, so it is in your interest to select your soundtrack carefully.

Research shows that music (Kaelan et al. 2018) can positively impact mood, enhance imagery, and prevent anxious reactions during a trip.[14]

Try to select music that you enjoy and that resonates with your current mood and your intention for the experience as these factors appear to have a positive effect on the therapeutic outcomes.

A consultation with a trained music therapist is also a worthy consideration.

CHECK IN

Immediately prior to your trip, check in with your feelings and emotions. Pause and ask, "How am I

14. Kaelen, Mendel et. al. 2018. "The hidden therapist: evidence for a central role of music in psychedelic therapy." *Psychopharmacology, 235(2)*: 505-519. doi.org/10.1007/s00213-017-4820-5

feeling? Energized? Tense? Fearful? Calm?"

One way to do this is to:

- Close your eyes.

- Take a few long, slow, deep breaths, inhaling through your nose and exhaling through your mouth.

- Begin to inhabit and identify with your physical body, consciously becoming aware of any emotions, pain, tension, comfort, etc.

- Start with physical sensations as a way to be present, and then move into the felt sense. Ask yourself, "What is the 'weather,' the general atmosphere, of my current state?"

- Take note of the first thoughts that come to mind.

If you're feeling tense or resistant, one way to help clear those feelings is to focus on the sensations of love, joy, safety, and connection starting in your heart and radiating throughout your body. Continue to pay attention to your breath. Take as much time as you need to bring your mind and body to a state of calm centeredness before you begin.

Depending on the depth and intensity of your planned experience, this may be difficult to do. It's okay and normal to begin a trip from a state of nervousness. So long as you follow the preparation process and are in a safe, comfortable setting, trust that you are ready.

Exploration:
What to do during your trip

Your willingness to surrender to the experience has been shown to directly affect the depth and quality of your psychedelic experience. To the extent that you feel safe and able, allow yourself to flow with the experience and go where it takes you. Try not to control the visions or emotions or feelings that come up. Rather, try to stay open; invite them and let them move through you like passing waves.

During a trip, thoughts, emotions, or insights will likely flow in a more abundant, unpredictable, and unfamiliar way. Growth comes from the realization that you are not your thoughts; you can decide how you internalize them and take them into your life. This is done by first letting them be there, inviting them in when you'd normally close or tighten, and observing them as an interested objective witness hoping to learn.

When visions or words or scenes come up that you feel compelled to capture and write down in the form of words, shapes, or doodles, we include space in the journal to record these.

Notes taken during a trip are invaluable insights into the experience and what it showed you for you to reflect on and remember for ongoing integration long after the trip ends.

Reflection:
What to do after your trip

CHECK IN

As you ease out of the experience and come back
into the room and your body, notice the emotions
and associated physical sensations that are present,
and write them all down. Again, be honest and don't
self-censor. All of your feelings are valid, regardless of
how silly or insignificant they may seem, and there is
valuable information in everything that emerges during
and after your trip.

Take your time, close your eyes, and breathe; observe
the residual as well as any new feelings, sensations, and
thoughts that come up.

You'll likely emerge with a wealth of new perspectives,
insights, and questions about yourself and the world.
At first, this may seem like a senseless jumble of
thoughts and visions swirling in your mind. Before
trying to make sense of it all, take the time to simply

notice them, like objects on a table or passing waves in the ocean.

Allowing yourself twenty to thirty minutes to meditate will help you start to process and encode the experience.

As Lama Surya Das writes in *Awakening the Buddha Within:* "We meditate in order to understand and directly perceive reality or truth—defined by the Buddha as 'clear seeing,' or 'seeing things as they are.' We meditate in order to wake up to what is, and thus arrive at the total immediacy and authenticity of life in this very present moment. That's the goal, and it is also the practice. Cultivating present, moment-by-moment awareness helps you come home to who you are and always have been."

If you have meditation recordings or an app that you find calming and helpful, lean on that, but it's not necessary. Meditation requires little; all you have to do is stop doing and just be. Sit with your current state; invite whatever is there to be felt and flow through you.

You may do this by finding a comfortable seat, closing your eyes, and beginning to connect to your breath. Feel the weight of your body on the earth and scan your awareness from the top of your head down your neck, chest, and belly and down your limbs, fingers, and toes. Then broaden awareness to your whole body resting on this earth. Feel the energy alive and tingling in and between every cell.

Grounding and returning awareness to your physical body will help the experience sit with you and begin to gel. Many of us are more mental than somatic. That is, we understand and make sense of emotions and experiences with our minds before our bodies. But our bodies have their own level of intelligence, often a deeper, more intuitive one than our minds (the human body evolved long before the frontal cortex, after all). Following a trip, your mind is returning from a unique and stimulating journey. Rooting it back to its physical home can offer a more calming effect than immediately trying to make sense of thoughts. Don't worry. There's plenty of time to do that later with the guided questions we include in the Trip Journal section.

RELEASE

Trips can be dream-like. It's easy to forget and lose the key insights our unconscious tried to tell us unless we record them while they're fresh. After completing your trip and taking some time to meditate and be with it, use the Trip Journal to release any and all thoughts that come to mind about the experience, in no formatted way, to act as a foundation to build on with a more guided reflection a day or two later.

BIO BREAK & CONNECT

Take some time to physically care for yourself, eat something light, and drink water. Stretch and move. It might feel good to go for a walk. Avoid negative or activating media. Try to maintain a calm environment for the rest of the day, perhaps with more meditation, nature, visually pleasing movies, writing, drawing, relaxation with a book, or early sleep.

If you have a friend, therapist, or loved one to call on, do this now. Even if you're not ready to talk through the experience, feeling support from someone who knows and cares for you can be hugely valuable in easing back into reality.

REFLECT

When you're ready, pick up your Trip Journal, review your intention and initial notes to take your mind back into the experience, and start responding to the guided questions we include.

Often, time allows for further reflection and processing, so know that realizations may continue to flow for days or even months. Come back as often as you need to review and add to your journal.

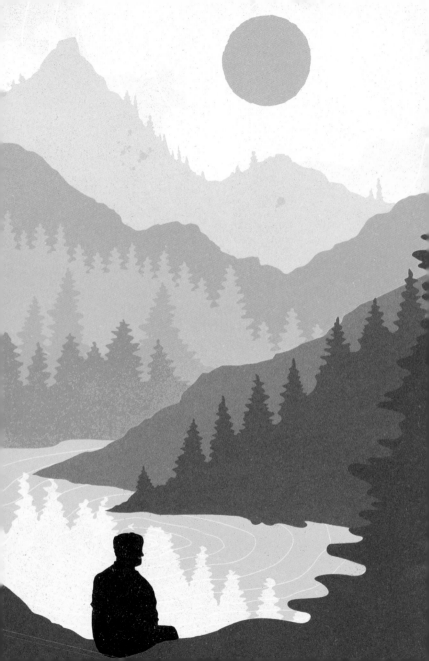

The universe is not
outside of you. Look inside
yourself; everything that you
want, you already are.

–RUMI

Integration:
Going beyond your trip

WHAT IS INTEGRATION?

Integration is the process by which you allow the experiences that occurred during your trip to translate to changes in your life. It is the act of turning insights into action that allows for sustained growth and change.

WHY IT MATTERS

Even though the physical aspects of your experience end soon after, research shows that the psychological effects of a trip can last for weeks after the actual psychedelic experience is over. New insights and questions may continue to emerge, so it's important to remain open as you reenter your daily life and to continue your internal work as the processing flows.

HOW TO DO IT

This guide is designed as a first step in the integration process by helping you record key aspects of your trip so as to start encoding them into your brain and psyche. It also acts as a record so that you can revisit your experiences with the benefit of time and further reflection, so come back to it as often as desired.

However, it is not designed to be your sole source of integration support. To fully integrate the experience, we also recommend speaking with a licensed psychologist or psychotherapist with experience in the work of integration.

Outside of therapy, there is no specific formula for integration, and there is no one-size-fits-all approach. Meditation, journaling (the *5-Minute Journal* by Intelligent Change Inc. is a great tool to start to implement and track your daily habits), and talking to friends can all be part of the process. Like your trip, the path to integration is personal, so feel free to experiment to find what works best for you.

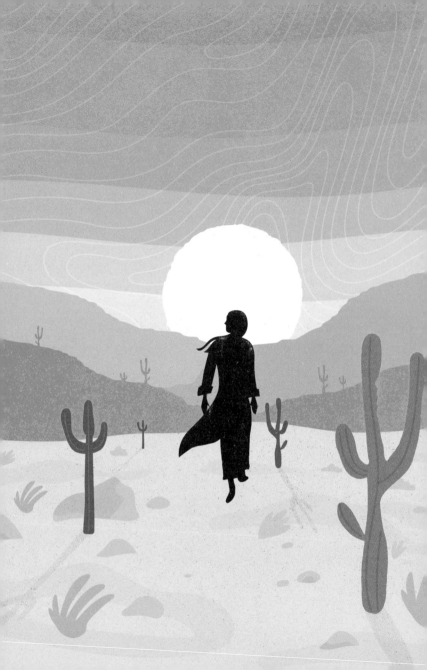

The Trip Journal

The real voyage of
discovery consists not in seeking
new landscapes, but in having
new eyes.

—MARCEL PROUST

Start date

Start time

Psychedelic

Dose

Location

How do you feel right now?

Check in with your mind and body before your trip:

- O Tense
- O Fearful
- O Calm
- O Energized
- O Empowered

- O Joyous
- O Loving
- O Inspired
- O Amused
- O Nostalgic

- O Satisfied
- O Angry
- O Sad
- O Tired
- O Confused

What is your intention?

What is the purpose or goal around which you want to center your experience?

This is your space. Write, draw, capture your experience in
any way that resonates with you.

*"If you want to fly, you have to give up everything
that weighs you down."* –TONI MORRISON

Date   Time

How do you feel right now?

Check in with your mind and body before your trip:

○ Tense	○ Joyous	○ Satisfied
○ Fearful	○ Loving	○ Angry
○ Calm	○ Inspired	○ Sad
○ Energized	○ Amused	○ Tired
○ Empowered	○ Nostalgic	○ Confused

Date   Time

How do you feel right now?

Check in with your mind and body before your trip:

O Tense	O Joyous	O Satisfied
O Fearful	O Loving	O Angry
O Calm	O Inspired	O Sad
O Energized	O Amused	O Tired
O Empowered	O Nostalgic	O Confused

What is coming up for you?

_____

_____

_____

_____

_____

_____

_____

_____

_____

_____

_____

Date   Time

How do you feel right now?

Check in with your mind and body before your trip:

- O Tense
- O Fearful
- O Calm
- O Energized
- O Empowered

- O Joyous
- O Loving
- O Inspired
- O Amused
- O Nostalgic

- O Satisfied
- O Angry
- O Sad
- O Tired
- O Confused

What is coming up for you?

Date   Time

How do you feel right now?

Check in with your mind and body before your trip:

O Tense	O Joyous	O Satisfied
O Fearful	O Loving	O Angry
O Calm	O Inspired	O Sad
O Energized	O Amused	O Tired
O Empowered	O Nostalgic	O Confused

What is coming up for you?

_____

_____

_____

_____

_____

_____

_____

_____

_____

_____

_____

Date   Time

How do you feel right now?

Check in with your mind and body before your trip:

  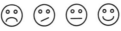

O Tense	O Joyous	O Satisfied
O Fearful	O Loving	O Angry
O Calm	O Inspired	O Sad
O Energized	O Amused	O Tired
O Empowered	O Nostalgic	O Confused

What is coming up for you?

_____

_____

_____

_____

_____

_____

_____

_____

_____

_____

_____

Date   Time

How do you feel right now?

Check in with your mind and body before your trip:

O Tense	O Joyous	O Satisfied
O Fearful	O Loving	O Angry
O Calm	O Inspired	O Sad
O Energized	O Amused	O Tired
O Empowered	O Nostalgic	O Confused

What is coming up for you?

_____

_____

_____

_____

_____

_____

_____

_____

_____

_____

_____

Date   Time

How do you feel right now?

Check in with your mind and body before your trip:

O Tense	O Joyous	O Satisfied
O Fearful	O Loving	O Angry
O Calm	O Inspired	O Sad
O Energized	O Amused	O Tired
O Empowered	O Nostalgic	O Confused

What is coming up for you?

_____

_____

_____

_____

_____

_____

_____

_____

_____

_____

_____

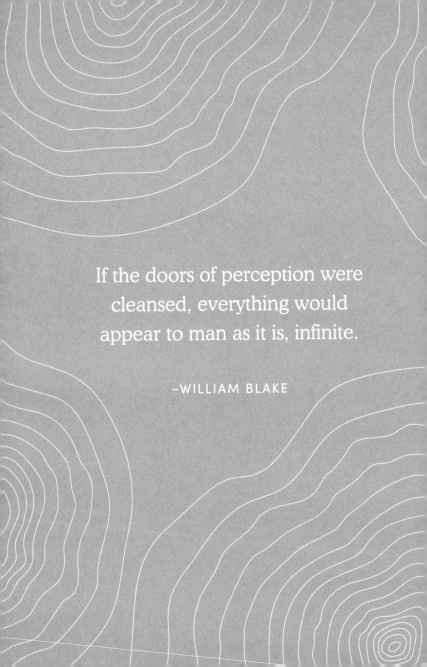

If the doors of perception were cleansed, everything would appear to man as it is, infinite.

–WILLIAM BLAKE

Start date

Start time

Psychedelic

Dose

Location

How do you feel right now?

Check in with your mind and body before your trip:

O Tense

O Joyous

O Satisfied

O Fearful

O Loving

O Angry

O Calm

O Inspired

O Sad

O Energized

O Amused

O Tired

O Empowered

O Nostalgic

O Confused

What is your intention?

What is the purpose or goal around which you want to

center your experience?

This is your space. Write, draw, capture your experience in
any way that resonates with you.

"In the journal I do not just express myself more openly than I could to any person; I create myself." –SUSAN SONTAG

Date   Time

How do you feel right now?

Check in with your mind and body before your trip:

O Tense	O Joyous	O Satisfied
O Fearful	O Loving	O Angry
O Calm	O Inspired	O Sad
O Energized	O Amused	O Tired
O Empowered	O Nostalgic	O Confused

Date   Time

How do you feel right now?

Check in with your mind and body before your trip:

O Tense	O Joyous	O Satisfied
O Fearful	O Loving	O Angry
O Calm	O Inspired	O Sad
O Energized	O Amused	O Tired
O Empowered	O Nostalgic	O Confused

What is coming up for you?

_____

_____

_____

_____

_____

_____

_____

_____

_____

_____

_____

Date   Time

How do you feel right now?

Check in with your mind and body before your trip:

O Tense	O Joyous	O Satisfied
O Fearful	O Loving	O Angry
O Calm	O Inspired	O Sad
O Energized	O Amused	O Tired
O Empowered	O Nostalgic	O Confused

What is coming up for you?

_____

_____

_____

_____

_____

_____

_____

_____

_____

_____

_____

Date   Time

How do you feel right now?

Check in with your mind and body before your trip:

○ Tense	○ Joyous	○ Satisfied
○ Fearful	○ Loving	○ Angry
○ Calm	○ Inspired	○ Sad
○ Energized	○ Amused	○ Tired
○ Empowered	○ Nostalgic	○ Confused

What is coming up for you?

_____

_____

_____

_____

_____

_____

_____

_____

_____

_____

_____

Date   Time

How do you feel right now?

Check in with your mind and body before your trip:

O Tense	O Joyous	O Satisfied
O Fearful	O Loving	O Angry
O Calm	O Inspired	O Sad
O Energized	O Amused	O Tired
O Empowered	O Nostalgic	O Confused

What is coming up for you?

_____

_____

_____

_____

_____

_____

_____

_____

_____

_____

_____

Date   Time

How do you feel right now?
Check in with your mind and body before your trip:

O Tense	O Joyous	O Satisfied
O Fearful	O Loving	O Angry
O Calm	O Inspired	O Sad
O Energized	O Amused	O Tired
O Empowered	O Nostalgic	O Confused

What is coming up for you?

_____

_____

_____

_____

_____

_____

_____

_____

_____

_____

_____

Date   Time

How do you feel right now?

Check in with your mind and body before your trip:

O Tense	O Joyous	O Satisfied
O Fearful	O Loving	O Angry
O Calm	O Inspired	O Sad
O Energized	O Amused	O Tired
O Empowered	O Nostalgic	O Confused

What is coming up for you?

_____

_____

_____

_____

_____

_____

_____

_____

_____

_____

_____

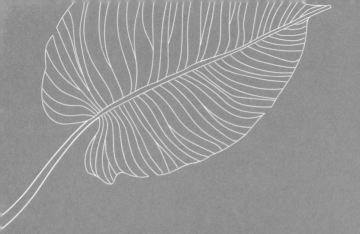

To be free, to come to terms
with our lives, we have to have a
direct experience of ourselves as
we really are, warts and all.

–MARK EPSTEIN

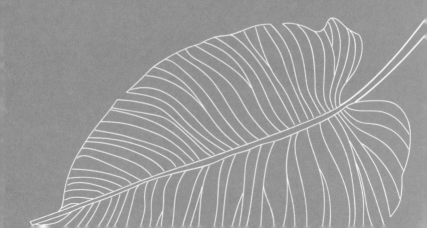

Start date   Start time

Psychedelic   Dose

Location

How do you feel right now?

Check in with your mind and body before your trip:

O Tense	O Joyous	O Satisfied
O Fearful	O Loving	O Angry
O Calm	O Inspired	O Sad
O Energized	O Amused	O Tired
O Empowered	O Nostalgic	O Confused

What is your intention?

What is the purpose or goal around which you want to

center your experience?

_____

_____

_____

_____

_____

_____

_____

This is your space. Write, draw, capture your experience in
any way that resonates with you.

"The only way we can change the way we feel is by becoming aware of our inner experience and learning to befriend what is going inside ourselves." –BESSEL VAN DER KOLK

Date   Time

How do you feel right now?
Check in with your mind and body before your trip:

O Tense	O Joyous	O Satisfied
O Fearful	O Loving	O Angry
O Calm	O Inspired	O Sad
O Energized	O Amused	O Tired
O Empowered	O Nostalgic	O Confused

Date   Time

How do you feel right now?
Check in with your mind and body before your trip:

O Tense	O Joyous	O Satisfied
O Fearful	O Loving	O Angry
O Calm	O Inspired	O Sad
O Energized	O Amused	O Tired
O Empowered	O Nostalgic	O Confused

What is coming up for you?

_____

_____

_____

_____

_____

_____

_____

_____

_____

_____

_____

_____

Date   Time

How do you feel right now?

Check in with your mind and body before your trip:

○ Tense	○ Joyous	○ Satisfied
○ Fearful	○ Loving	○ Angry
○ Calm	○ Inspired	○ Sad
○ Energized	○ Amused	○ Tired
○ Empowered	○ Nostalgic	○ Confused

What is coming up for you?

_____

_____

_____

_____

_____

_____

_____

_____

_____

_____

_____

Date   Time

How do you feel right now?

Check in with your mind and body before your trip:

O Tense	O Joyous	O Satisfied
O Fearful	O Loving	O Angry
O Calm	O Inspired	O Sad
O Energized	O Amused	O Tired
O Empowered	O Nostalgic	O Confused

What is coming up for you?

_____

_____

_____

_____

_____

_____

_____

_____

_____

_____

Date   Time

How do you feel right now?

Check in with your mind and body before your trip:

O Tense   O Joyous   O Satisfied
O Fearful   O Loving   O Angry
O Calm   O Inspired   O Sad
O Energized   O Amused   O Tired
O Empowered   O Nostalgic   O Confused

What is coming up for you?

_____

_____

_____

_____

_____

_____

_____

_____

_____

_____

_____

Date   Time

How do you feel right now?

Check in with your mind and body before your trip:

O Tense	O Joyous	O Satisfied
O Fearful	O Loving	O Angry
O Calm	O Inspired	O Sad
O Energized	O Amused	O Tired
O Empowered	O Nostalgic	O Confused

What is coming up for you?

_____

_____

_____

_____

_____

_____

_____

_____

_____

_____

_____

Date   Time

How do you feel right now?

Check in with your mind and body before your trip:

O Tense	O Joyous	O Satisfied
O Fearful	O Loving	O Angry
O Calm	O Inspired	O Sad
O Energized	O Amused	O Tired
O Empowered	O Nostalgic	O Confused

What is coming up for you?

_____

_____

_____

_____

_____

_____

_____

_____

_____

_____

_____

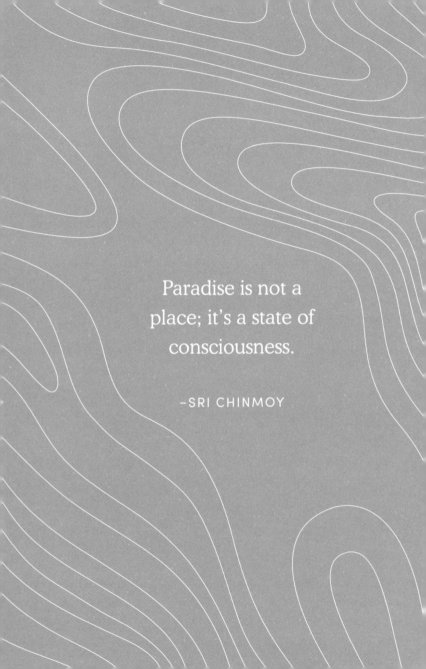

Paradise is not a place; it's a state of consciousness.

–SRI CHINMOY

Start date

Start time

Psychedelic

Dose

Location

How do you feel right now?

Check in with your mind and body before your trip:

O Tense	O Joyous	O Satisfied
O Fearful	O Loving	O Angry
O Calm	O Inspired	O Sad
O Energized	O Amused	O Tired
O Empowered	O Nostalgic	O Confused

What is your intention?

What is the purpose or goal around which you want to

center your experience?

This is your space. Write, draw, capture your experience in any way that resonates with you.

"Wherever you go, there you are."
–JON KABAT-ZINN

Date   Time

How do you feel right now?

Check in with your mind and body before your trip:

O Tense	O Joyous	O Satisfied
O Fearful	O Loving	O Angry
O Calm	O Inspired	O Sad
O Energized	O Amused	O Tired
O Empowered	O Nostalgic	O Confused

Date   Time

How do you feel right now?

Check in with your mind and body before your trip:

  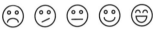

O Tense	O Joyous	O Satisfied
O Fearful	O Loving	O Angry
O Calm	O Inspired	O Sad
O Energized	O Amused	O Tired
O Empowered	O Nostalgic	O Confused

What is coming up for you?

_____

_____

_____

_____

_____

_____

_____

_____

_____

_____

Date   Time

How do you feel right now?

Check in with your mind and body before your trip:

O Tense	O Joyous	O Satisfied
O Fearful	O Loving	O Angry
O Calm	O Inspired	O Sad
O Energized	O Amused	O Tired
O Empowered	O Nostalgic	O Confused

What is coming up for you?

_____

_____

_____

_____

_____

_____

_____

_____

_____

_____

Date   Time

How do you feel right now?

Check in with your mind and body before your trip:

O Tense	O Joyous	O Satisfied
O Fearful	O Loving	O Angry
O Calm	O Inspired	O Sad
O Energized	O Amused	O Tired
O Empowered	O Nostalgic	O Confused

What is coming up for you?

_____

_____

_____

_____

_____

_____

_____

_____

_____

_____

_____

Date   Time

How do you feel right now?

Check in with your mind and body before your trip:

O Tense	O Joyous	O Satisfied
O Fearful	O Loving	O Angry
O Calm	O Inspired	O Sad
O Energized	O Amused	O Tired
O Empowered	O Nostalgic	O Confused

What is coming up for you?

_____

_____

_____

_____

_____

_____

_____

_____

_____

_____

_____

Date   Time

How do you feel right now?

Check in with your mind and body before your trip:

O Tense	O Joyous	O Satisfied
O Fearful	O Loving	O Angry
O Calm	O Inspired	O Sad
O Energized	O Amused	O Tired
O Empowered	O Nostalgic	O Confused

What is coming up for you?

_____

_____

_____

_____

_____

_____

_____

_____

_____

_____

_____

Date   Time

How do you feel right now?

Check in with your mind and body before your trip:

O Tense	O Joyous	O Satisfied
O Fearful	O Loving	O Angry
O Calm	O Inspired	O Sad
O Energized	O Amused	O Tired
O Empowered	O Nostalgic	O Confused

What is coming up for you?

_____

_____

_____

_____

_____

_____

_____

_____

_____

_____

_____

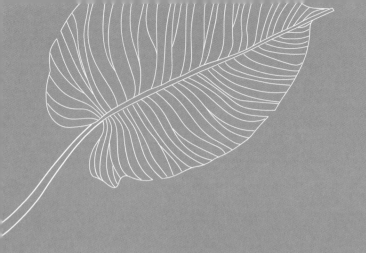

It takes enormous trust and courage to allow yourself to remember.

−BESSEL VAN DER KOLK

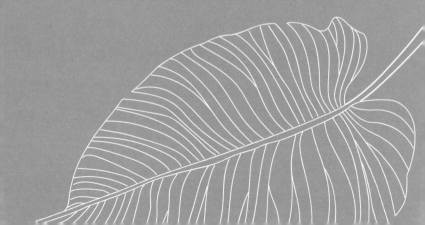

Start date · · · · · · · · · · · Start time

Psychedelic · · · · · · · · · · · Dose

Location · · · · · · · · · · ·

How do you feel right now?

Check in with your mind and body before your trip:

O Tense
O Fearful
O Calm
O Energized
O Empowered

O Joyous
O Loving
O Inspired
O Amused
O Nostalgic

O Satisfied
O Angry
O Sad
O Tired
O Confused

What is your intention?

What is the purpose or goal around which you want to

center your experience?

_____

_____

_____

_____

_____

_____

_____

_____

This is your space. Write, draw, capture your experience in any way that resonates with you.

"The picture we present to ourselves of who we think we ought to be obscures who we really are." –MARK EPSTEIN

Date   Time

How do you feel right now?

Check in with your mind and body before your trip:

O Tense	O Joyous	O Satisfied
O Fearful	O Loving	O Angry
O Calm	O Inspired	O Sad
O Energized	O Amused	O Tired
O Empowered	O Nostalgic	O Confused

Date   Time

How do you feel right now?

Check in with your mind and body before your trip:

O Tense	O Joyous	O Satisfied
O Fearful	O Loving	O Angry
O Calm	O Inspired	O Sad
O Energized	O Amused	O Tired
O Empowered	O Nostalgic	O Confused

What is coming up for you?

_____

_____

_____

_____

_____

_____

_____

_____

_____

_____

_____

Date   Time

How do you feel right now?

Check in with your mind and body before your trip:

O Tense	O Joyous	O Satisfied
O Fearful	O Loving	O Angry
O Calm	O Inspired	O Sad
O Energized	O Amused	O Tired
O Empowered	O Nostalgic	O Confused

What is coming up for you?

_____

_____

_____

_____

_____

_____

_____

_____

_____

_____

_____

Date   Time

How do you feel right now?

Check in with your mind and body before your trip:

○ Tense	○ Joyous	○ Satisfied
○ Fearful	○ Loving	○ Angry
○ Calm	○ Inspired	○ Sad
○ Energized	○ Amused	○ Tired
○ Empowered	○ Nostalgic	○ Confused

What is coming up for you?

_____

_____

_____

_____

_____

_____

_____

_____

_____

_____

_____

Date   Time

How do you feel right now?

Check in with your mind and body before your trip:

O Tense	O Joyous	O Satisfied
O Fearful	O Loving	O Angry
O Calm	O Inspired	O Sad
O Energized	O Amused	O Tired
O Empowered	O Nostalgic	O Confused

What is coming up for you?

_____

_____

_____

_____

_____

_____

_____

_____

_____

_____

_____

Date   Time

How do you feel right now?

Check in with your mind and body before your trip:

O Tense	O Joyous	O Satisfied
O Fearful	O Loving	O Angry
O Calm	O Inspired	O Sad
O Energized	O Amused	O Tired
O Empowered	O Nostalgic	O Confused

What is coming up for you?

_____

_____

_____

_____

_____

_____

_____

_____

_____

_____

_____

Date   Time

How do you feel right now?

Check in with your mind and body before your trip:

O Tense	O Joyous	O Satisfied
O Fearful	O Loving	O Angry
O Calm	O Inspired	O Sad
O Energized	O Amused	O Tired
O Empowered	O Nostalgic	O Confused

What is coming up for you?

_____

_____

_____

_____

_____

_____

_____

_____

_____

_____

_____

Awakening does not mean
a change in difficulty, it means
a change in how those
difficulties are met.

—MARK EPSTEIN

Start date   Start time

Psychedelic   Dose

Location

How do you feel right now?

Check in with your mind and body before your trip:

O Tense	O Joyous	O Satisfied
O Fearful	O Loving	O Angry
O Calm	O Inspired	O Sad
O Energized	O Amused	O Tired
O Empowered	O Nostalgic	O Confused

What is your intention?

What is the purpose or goal around which you want to

center your experience?

This is your space. Write, draw, capture your experience in any way that resonates with you.

"I write because I don't know what I think until I read what I say."
—FLANNERY O'CONNOR

Date   Time

How do you feel right now?

Check in with your mind and body before your trip:

○ Tense	○ Joyous	○ Satisfied
○ Fearful	○ Loving	○ Angry
○ Calm	○ Inspired	○ Sad
○ Energized	○ Amused	○ Tired
○ Empowered	○ Nostalgic	○ Confused

_____

_____

_____

_____

_____

_____

_____

_____

_____

_____

Date   Time

How do you feel right now?

Check in with your mind and body before your trip:

O Tense	O Joyous	O Satisfied
O Fearful	O Loving	O Angry
O Calm	O Inspired	O Sad
O Energized	O Amused	O Tired
O Empowered	O Nostalgic	O Confused

What is coming up for you?

_____

_____

_____

_____

_____

_____

_____

_____

_____

_____

_____

Date   Time

How do you feel right now?

Check in with your mind and body before your trip:

O Tense	O Joyous	O Satisfied
O Fearful	O Loving	O Angry
O Calm	O Inspired	O Sad
O Energized	O Amused	O Tired
O Empowered	O Nostalgic	O Confused

What is coming up for you?

_____

_____

_____

_____

_____

_____

_____

_____

_____

_____

_____

Date   Time

How do you feel right now?

Check in with your mind and body before your trip:

O Tense   O Joyous   O Satisfied
O Fearful   O Loving   O Angry
O Calm   O Inspired   O Sad
O Energized   O Amused   O Tired
O Empowered   O Nostalgic   O Confused

What is coming up for you?

_____

_____

_____

_____

_____

_____

_____

_____

_____

_____

_____

Date   Time

How do you feel right now?

Check in with your mind and body before your trip:

O Tense	O Joyous	O Satisfied
O Fearful	O Loving	O Angry
O Calm	O Inspired	O Sad
O Energized	O Amused	O Tired
O Empowered	O Nostalgic	O Confused

What is coming up for you?

Date   Time

How do you feel right now?

Check in with your mind and body before your trip:

O Tense	O Joyous	O Satisfied
O Fearful	O Loving	O Angry
O Calm	O Inspired	O Sad
O Energized	O Amused	O Tired
O Empowered	O Nostalgic	O Confused

What is coming up for you?

_____

_____

_____

_____

_____

_____

_____

_____

_____

_____

_____

Date   Time

How do you feel right now?

Check in with your mind and body before your trip:

O Tense	O Joyous	O Satisfied
O Fearful	O Loving	O Angry
O Calm	O Inspired	O Sad
O Energized	O Amused	O Tired
O Empowered	O Nostalgic	O Confused

What is coming up for you?

_____

_____

_____

_____

_____

_____

_____

_____

_____

_____

When I let go of what I am,
I become what I might be.

—LAO TZU

Start date

Start time

Psychedelic

Dose

Location

How do you feel right now?

Check in with your mind and body before your trip:

- O Tense
- O Fearful
- O Calm
- O Energized
- O Empowered

- O Joyous
- O Loving
- O Inspired
- O Amused
- O Nostalgic

- O Satisfied
- O Angry
- O Sad
- O Tired
- O Confused

What is your intention?

What is the purpose or goal around which you want to

center your experience?

This is your space. Write, draw, capture your experience in any way that resonates with you.

"The wound is the place where the light enters you."

–RUMI

Date   Time

How do you feel right now?

Check in with your mind and body before your trip:

O Tense	O Joyous	O Satisfied
O Fearful	O Loving	O Angry
O Calm	O Inspired	O Sad
O Energized	O Amused	O Tired
O Empowered	O Nostalgic	O Confused

Date   Time

How do you feel right now?

Check in with your mind and body before your trip:

O Tense	O Joyous	O Satisfied
O Fearful	O Loving	O Angry
O Calm	O Inspired	O Sad
O Energized	O Amused	O Tired
O Empowered	O Nostalgic	O Confused

What is coming up for you?

_____

_____

_____

_____

_____

_____

_____

_____

_____

_____

_____

Date   Time

How do you feel right now?

Check in with your mind and body before your trip:

O Tense	O Joyous	O Satisfied
O Fearful	O Loving	O Angry
O Calm	O Inspired	O Sad
O Energized	O Amused	O Tired
O Empowered	O Nostalgic	O Confused

What is coming up for you?

_____

_____

_____

_____

_____

_____

_____

_____

_____

_____

Date   Time

How do you feel right now?

Check in with your mind and body before your trip:

O Tense   O Joyous   O Satisfied

O Fearful   O Loving   O Angry

O Calm   O Inspired   O Sad

O Energized   O Amused   O Tired

O Empowered   O Nostalgic   O Confused

What is coming up for you?

Date   Time

How do you feel right now?

Check in with your mind and body before your trip:

  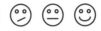

O Tense	O Joyous	O Satisfied
O Fearful	O Loving	O Angry
O Calm	O Inspired	O Sad
O Energized	O Amused	O Tired
O Empowered	O Nostalgic	O Confused

What is coming up for you?

_____

_____

_____

_____

_____

_____

_____

_____

_____

_____

_____

_____

Date   Time

How do you feel right now?

Check in with your mind and body before your trip:

O Tense	O Joyous	O Satisfied
O Fearful	O Loving	O Angry
O Calm	O Inspired	O Sad
O Energized	O Amused	O Tired
O Empowered	O Nostalgic	O Confused

What is coming up for you?

_____

_____

_____

_____

_____

_____

_____

_____

_____

_____

_____

Date   Time

How do you feel right now?

Check in with your mind and body before your trip:

  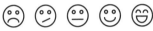

O Tense	O Joyous	O Satisfied
O Fearful	O Loving	O Angry
O Calm	O Inspired	O Sad
O Energized	O Amused	O Tired
O Empowered	O Nostalgic	O Confused

What is coming up for you?

_____

_____

_____

_____

_____

_____

_____

_____

_____

_____

_____

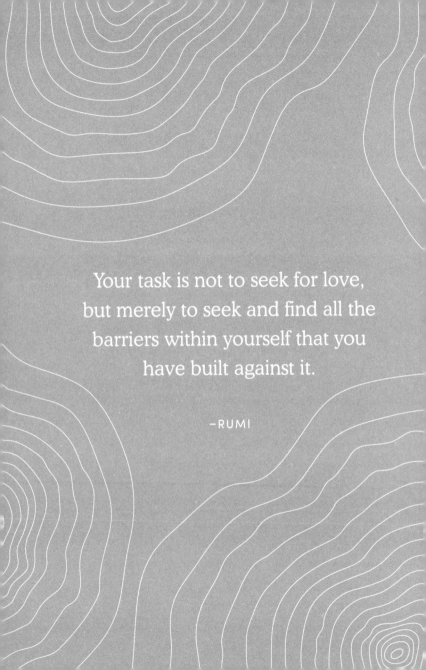

Your task is not to seek for love,
but merely to seek and find all the
barriers within yourself that you
have built against it.

—RUMI

Start date   Start time

Psychedelic   Dose

Location

How do you feel right now?

Check in with your mind and body before your trip:

O Tense	O Joyous	O Satisfied
O Fearful	O Loving	O Angry
O Calm	O Inspired	O Sad
O Energized	O Amused	O Tired
O Empowered	O Nostalgic	O Confused

What is your intention?

What is the purpose or goal around which you want to

center your experience?

This is your space. Write, draw, capture your experience in any way that resonates with you.

"There is nothing good nor bad, but thinking makes it so."
—SHAKESPEARE

Date   Time

How do you feel right now?

Check in with your mind and body before your trip:

O Tense	O Joyous	O Satisfied
O Fearful	O Loving	O Angry
O Calm	O Inspired	O Sad
O Energized	O Amused	O Tired
O Empowered	O Nostalgic	O Confused

_____

_____

_____

_____

_____

_____

_____

_____

_____

_____

_____

Date   Time

How do you feel right now?

Check in with your mind and body before your trip:

O Tense	O Joyous	O Satisfied
O Fearful	O Loving	O Angry
O Calm	O Inspired	O Sad
O Energized	O Amused	O Tired
O Empowered	O Nostalgic	O Confused

What is coming up for you?

_____

_____

_____

_____

_____

_____

_____

_____

_____

_____

_____

Date   Time

How do you feel right now?

Check in with your mind and body before your trip:

O Tense	O Joyous	O Satisfied
O Fearful	O Loving	O Angry
O Calm	O Inspired	O Sad
O Energized	O Amused	O Tired
O Empowered	O Nostalgic	O Confused

What is coming up for you?

_____

_____

_____

_____

_____

_____

_____

_____

_____

_____

_____

Date   Time

How do you feel right now?

Check in with your mind and body before your trip:

O Tense	O Joyous	O Satisfied
O Fearful	O Loving	O Angry
O Calm	O Inspired	O Sad
O Energized	O Amused	O Tired
O Empowered	O Nostalgic	O Confused

What is coming up for you?

_____

_____

_____

_____

_____

_____

_____

_____

_____

_____

_____

Date   Time

How do you feel right now?

Check in with your mind and body before your trip:

O Tense	O Joyous	O Satisfied
O Fearful	O Loving	O Angry
O Calm	O Inspired	O Sad
O Energized	O Amused	O Tired
O Empowered	O Nostalgic	O Confused

What is coming up for you?

_____

_____

_____

_____

_____

_____

_____

_____

_____

_____

_____

Date   Time

How do you feel right now?
Check in with your mind and body before your trip:

O Tense	O Joyous	O Satisfied
O Fearful	O Loving	O Angry
O Calm	O Inspired	O Sad
O Energized	O Amused	O Tired
O Empowered	O Nostalgic	O Confused

What is coming up for you?

_____

_____

_____

_____

_____

_____

_____

_____

_____

_____

Date   Time

How do you feel right now?

Check in with your mind and body before your trip:

O Tense	O Joyous	O Satisfied
O Fearful	O Loving	O Angry
O Calm	O Inspired	O Sad
O Energized	O Amused	O Tired
O Empowered	O Nostalgic	O Confused

What is coming up for you?

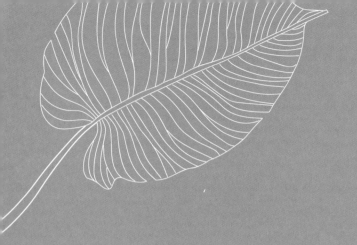

Fear is a natural reaction to
moving closer to the truth.

–PEMA CHÖDRÖN

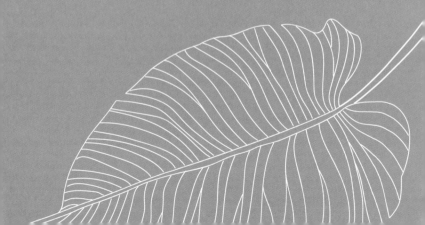

Start date

Start time

Psychedelic

Dose

Location

How do you feel right now?

Check in with your mind and body before your trip:

O Tense	O Joyous	O Satisfied
O Fearful	O Loving	O Angry
O Calm	O Inspired	O Sad
O Energized	O Amused	O Tired
O Empowered	O Nostalgic	O Confused

What is your intention?

What is the purpose or goal around which you want to

center your experience?

This is your space. Write, draw, capture your experience in
any way that resonates with you.

"We are healed of a suffering only by experiencing it to the full."

-MARCEL PROUST

Date   Time

How do you feel right now?

Check in with your mind and body before your trip:

O Tense	O Joyous	O Satisfied
O Fearful	O Loving	O Angry
O Calm	O Inspired	O Sad
O Energized	O Amused	O Tired
O Empowered	O Nostalgic	O Confused

Date   Time

How do you feel right now?

Check in with your mind and body before your trip:

O Tense	O Joyous	O Satisfied
O Fearful	O Loving	O Angry
O Calm	O Inspired	O Sad
O Energized	O Amused	O Tired
O Empowered	O Nostalgic	O Confused

What is coming up for you?

_____

_____

_____

_____

_____

_____

_____

_____

_____

_____

_____

Date   Time

How do you feel right now?

Check in with your mind and body before your trip:

O Tense	O Joyous	O Satisfied
O Fearful	O Loving	O Angry
O Calm	O Inspired	O Sad
O Energized	O Amused	O Tired
O Empowered	O Nostalgic	O Confused

What is coming up for you?

_____

_____

_____

_____

_____

_____

_____

_____

_____

_____

Date   Time

How do you feel right now?

Check in with your mind and body before your trip:

O Tense	O Joyous	O Satisfied
O Fearful	O Loving	O Angry
O Calm	O Inspired	O Sad
O Energized	O Amused	O Tired
O Empowered	O Nostalgic	O Confused

What is coming up for you?

_____

_____

_____

_____

_____

_____

_____

_____

_____

_____

_____

Date   Time

How do you feel right now?
Check in with your mind and body before your trip:

O Tense	O Joyous	O Satisfied
O Fearful	O Loving	O Angry
O Calm	O Inspired	O Sad
O Energized	O Amused	O Tired
O Empowered	O Nostalgic	O Confused

What is coming up for you?

_____

_____

_____

_____

_____

_____

_____

_____

_____

_____

_____

Date   Time

How do you feel right now?

Check in with your mind and body before your trip:

O Tense	O Joyous	O Satisfied
O Fearful	O Loving	O Angry
O Calm	O Inspired	O Sad
O Energized	O Amused	O Tired
O Empowered	O Nostalgic	O Confused

What is coming up for you?

_____

_____

_____

_____

_____

_____

_____

_____

_____

_____

_____

Date   Time

How do you feel right now?

Check in with your mind and body before your trip:

O Tense	O Joyous	O Satisfied
O Fearful	O Loving	O Angry
O Calm	O Inspired	O Sad
O Energized	O Amused	O Tired
O Empowered	O Nostalgic	O Confused

What is coming up for you?

_____

_____

_____

_____

_____

_____

_____

_____

_____

_____

_____

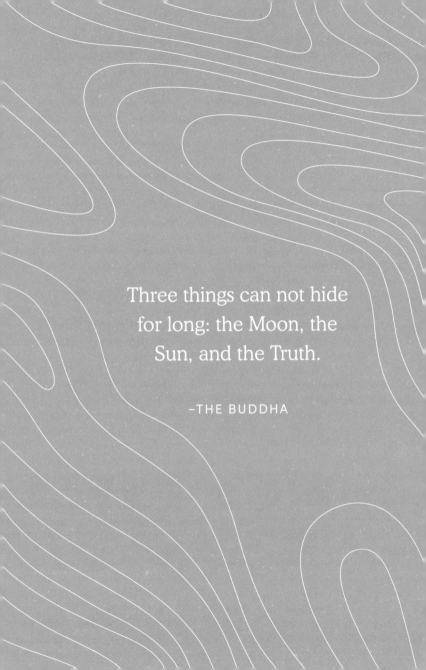

Three things can not hide
for long: the Moon, the
Sun, and the Truth.

–THE BUDDHA

Start date   Start time

Psychedelic   Dose

Location

How do you feel right now?

Check in with your mind and body before your trip:

😦 😕 😐 🙂 😄

O Tense   O Joyous   O Satisfied
O Fearful   O Loving   O Angry
O Calm   O Inspired   O Sad
O Energized   O Amused   O Tired
O Empowered   O Nostalgic   O Confused

What is your intention?

What is the purpose or goal around which you want to

center your experience?

_____

_____

_____

_____

_____

_____

_____

_____

This is your space. Write, draw, capture your experience in any way that resonates with you.

"Watch, witness. Your body is not you; your mind is not you. You are just a pure witness." -OSHO

Date   Time

How do you feel right now?
Check in with your mind and body before your trip:

O Tense	O Joyous	O Satisfied
O Fearful	O Loving	O Angry
O Calm	O Inspired	O Sad
O Energized	O Amused	O Tired
O Empowered	O Nostalgic	O Confused

Date   Time

How do you feel right now?

Check in with your mind and body before your trip:

O Tense	O Joyous	O Satisfied
O Fearful	O Loving	O Angry
O Calm	O Inspired	O Sad
O Energized	O Amused	O Tired
O Empowered	O Nostalgic	O Confused

What is coming up for you?

_____

_____

_____

_____

_____

_____

_____

_____

_____

_____

_____

Date   Time

How do you feel right now?

Check in with your mind and body before your trip:

O Tense	O Joyous	O Satisfied
O Fearful	O Loving	O Angry
O Calm	O Inspired	O Sad
O Energized	O Amused	O Tired
O Empowered	O Nostalgic	O Confused

What is coming up for you?

_____

_____

_____

_____

_____

_____

_____

_____

_____

_____

_____

Date   Time

How do you feel right now?

Check in with your mind and body before your trip:

O Tense	O Joyous	O Satisfied
O Fearful	O Loving	O Angry
O Calm	O Inspired	O Sad
O Energized	O Amused	O Tired
O Empowered	O Nostalgic	O Confused

What is coming up for you?

_____

_____

_____

_____

_____

_____

_____

_____

_____

_____

Date   Time

How do you feel right now?

Check in with your mind and body before your trip:

O Tense	O Joyous	O Satisfied
O Fearful	O Loving	O Angry
O Calm	O Inspired	O Sad
O Energized	O Amused	O Tired
O Empowered	O Nostalgic	O Confused

What is coming up for you?

_____

_____

_____

_____

_____

_____

_____

_____

_____

_____

_____

Date   Time

How do you feel right now?

Check in with your mind and body before your trip:

O Tense	O Joyous	O Satisfied
O Fearful	O Loving	O Angry
O Calm	O Inspired	O Sad
O Energized	O Amused	O Tired
O Empowered	O Nostalgic	O Confused

What is coming up for you?

_____

_____

_____

_____

_____

_____

_____

_____

_____

_____

_____

Date   Time

How do you feel right now?

Check in with your mind and body before your trip:

O Tense	O Joyous	O Satisfied
O Fearful	O Loving	O Angry
O Calm	O Inspired	O Sad
O Energized	O Amused	O Tired
O Empowered	O Nostalgic	O Confused

What is coming up for you?

_____

_____

_____

_____

_____

_____

_____

_____

_____

_____

Rest & Reset

You've come a long way. Take a deep breath and congratulate yourself for completing and reflecting on ten journeys inward. Thank you for allowing us to guide you along this courageous, vulnerable path. May your insights continue to flow; may you be well and thrive in this dance that is life.

Let the journeys continue by visiting tripjournal.co to download our app or order a new journal.